The Cosmetic Label Snob

The GreenSistah™'s Guide to

100 Nasty Ingredients You Should Avoid in Your

Cosmetics

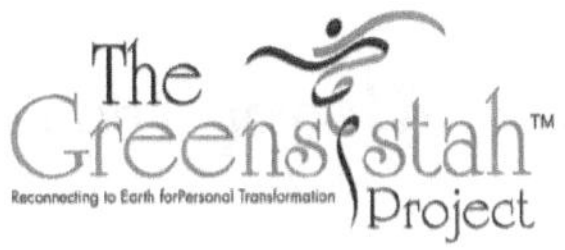

A GreenSistah™ Publication

Hampton, Virginia

greensistah.com

Offerings of Gratitude

I am grateful beyond words for the blessing of the knowledge shared in this work.

My gratitude to Vernell, my incredible daughter. Your editorial support, motivation, and patience throughout this process is immensely appreciated. You are my rock, and I love you.

I am grateful for my teachers throughout the years.

To my friends and family that encouraged me.

To you the reader, I am grateful for your purchase.

"Chemicals have replaced bacteria and viruses as the main threat to health. The diseases of the 1900's and into the 21st century are diseases of chemical origin."

-Dr. Dick Irwin, Toxicologist, Texas A&M University

The above quote is why I wrote this book. It led me to the horrible discovery of the dangers of the chemicals in cosmetic and personal care product.

You should know the dangers of these chemicals so that you can make educated choices about what you use on your hair, skin, and nails.

Willette (aka) The GreenSistah™

Introduction

A cosmetic label snob is an individual that insists on the best cosmetic and body care products available. The product has to offer the best ingredients nature has to offer and free of potentially toxic chemical or other harmful components. Furthermore, the product has to be formulated with elements historically proven effective for purposes intended. A cosmetic label snob is not impressed with celebrity endorsements, pretty labels, alluring synthetic fragrances, or savvy marketing campaigns. The ingredients on the label have to pass the test to go home with a Cosmetic Label Snob.

Why is that important? There are more than 10,500 chemicals cosmetic manufacturers are free to use in the products marketed for use on your hair skin and nails. According to the Environmental Working Group (EWG), only 11% have been assessed for safety by the FDA. Moreover, if you are like most women, you probably use more than 13 different cosmetic products every day like hairspray, deodorant, lipstick, foundation, toothpaste, shaving cream, moisturizers, and the list goes on. Your daily hygiene routine may be exposing you to more than 160 chemicals daily.   More common than you may expect, there is:

- **lead in your lipstick**

- **formaldehyde in baby shampoo**

- **reproductive toxins in hair relaxers**

- **carcinogens in hair dyes**

- **mercury in mascara**

- **agent orange in antibacterial soaps**

- **aluminum in antiperspirants**

- **allergens in perfumes**

- **oxybenzone in 60 percent of sunscreens**

- **endocrine disruptors in more than 13,000 cosmetics**

Even more disturbing, if you are an African -American women, you bear a disproportionate burden of the chemicals in cosmetics when compared to other

demographics.   Products sold to women of color

 such as skin lighteners, hair straighteners, and texturizers

and hair dyes contain reproductive toxins, carcinogens,

allergens, and immune system toxins. The barrage of

chemicals in your cosmetics, and personal care products

are taking its toll on health and life, and its time you

become aware. Knowledge is empowering, moreover,

when it comes to the chemicals in your cosmetics,

awareness knowledge, and application of that knowledge

can protect your health and save your life.

My goal in offering this work is to create awareness that

will empower you to your transformation to a healthier

personal care routine. I have listed 100 chemicals that

may be in your cosmetics and how they can impact your

health. My prayer is that as a result of your awareness,

you will begin to read labels, define ingredients, and

make safe and healthy choices. Furthermore, you will use

this work as a starting point to doing your research, teach

your children, and become a part of the necessary change.

The Beginning

My journey began with my hair in 1989. Once I discovered the danger I could be facing from the chemicals in my cosmetics, I decided that my addiction to the chemical relaxer had to end. Besides, the relaxer left my hair dry and brittle, and it never looked good on me. Braids were starting to be popular, so I jumped on board, and it seemed to do the trick for me. My style would hold up until I went back to the salon, and my hair started growing and thickening up.

As I became increasingly determined to live a healthier, more natural lifestyle, I started to question the synthetic hair I was using for the braids. My research revealed that the hair is a combination of plastics and other synthetics harmful to my scalp. I learned that using the extensions may lead to harmful bacteria and fungus passing onto my scalp. With that knowledge, I had to take my natural hair journey a step further. I ditched the braids and starting locking my hair in 1999. I'm currently on my third set of locs, two times traditional and presently rocking the Sisterlocks, and there is no going back.

It's a beautiful sight to see other Black women rock and embrace their natural hair and embrace a natural lifestyle overall, including skincare, and diet. It's a movement that appears to be gaining momentum at rocket speed. In every demographic, from doctors to lawyers, corporate

executives, administrative workers, and even the U.S.

military, Black women are ditching relaxer kits for braids,

locs, twist outs, blowouts, Bantu knots, puffs and afros at

stunning rates.

It appears that the natural hair movement is the genesis of

a "Self-Love" revolution.

The Cosmetic Label Snob Emerges!

As I became more determined to live a healthier life, my natural journey became more than just a hairstyle. I became committed to using only products that contained safe, clean, and healthy ingredients in my self-care routine.

 Determined to find the products with the absolute best ingredients without compromise, I visited health food stores. I found no natural formulations specifically for my textured curly hair. Some products may have posted

an acceptable component on the front of the label,
however, turning the name around there would be a slew
of undesirable ingredients. On the other hand, the
formulation may not have been sufficient for my needs.
As I searched, if there was even one ingredient that was
unhealthy or synthetic, it was no deal. I'm not buying it.

Frustrated with the limited choices, I decided that I would
have to make it myself and did just that. I dreamed up the
ingredients one night and from there created a product
which I named Sheajoba®. It was a base of shea butter
and jojoba with essential oils and other plant ingredients.
I used it on my hair, skin, and nails cause, after all, it's the
same stuff, and it worked. My hair stopped breaking, the

ash disappeared, and I was glowing from head to toe. I began sharing it with friends and family, and when they started coming back for seconds, I started charging them, and they paid. That was the start of my company, "Pretty Natural." Sheajoba™ was one of the first natural products formulated for Black women sold in Whole Foods and Mom's Organic Market.

The Nasty 100

As the following list will reveal, many of the ingredients that make up the products you use in your everyday hygiene and beauty routine are far from being clean and beautiful. U. S. researchers report that one in eight of the 10,500 chemicals used in personal care products is industrial chemicals, including carcinogens, pesticides, reproductive toxins, and hormone disruptors.

In many of the products you use on your hair, skin, and nails, you find formulations that include plasticizers (chemicals that keep concrete soft). You will also find degreasers (used to keep oil off auto parts), and surfactants (they reduce surface tension in water, like in paint and inks). Can you imagine what these chemicals can do to your body and the environment?

1. Acrylics (Acrylic Acid Ethyl Ester, Ethyl Acrylate, Methacrylic Acid, Methyl Methacrylic)

Used in artificial nail products and found in the adhesive for fake nails and eyelashes. Health concerns include cancer, developmental and reproductive toxicity organ system toxicity; may cause cellular and neurological damage and irritation.

2. Aluminum (Pure Aluminum Powder, Aluminum flake)

Used as a cosmetic colorant this ingredient scores 4-9 on EWG's Skin Deep Database. Health concerns include allergies and immunotoxicity. Neurotoxicity; enhanced skin absorption; organ system toxicity.

3. Aluminum Chloride (Aluminum Trichloride)

Used on the skin to decrease sweat and odor, widely used in deodorants, used in astringents. Health concerns include neurotoxins and links

to Alzheimer's allergies and immune system
disorders.

4. Aluminum Hydrochloride

Used in deodorants, antiperspirants, cosmetic
astringents. Health concerns include organ
system toxicity.

5. Aluminum Oxide

Used as a thickening and anti-caking agent, it
is found in foundations, blush, and lipstick.
Health concerns around this chemical include
toxic to nervous system and respiratory irritant.

6. Ammonium Persulfate

Used in hair bleaches and skin lighteners

Health concerns include organ system toxicity,

allergen, and skin irritant

7. Amyl Acetate (acetic acid)

A toxic solvent used in nail polish, acts as a

central nervous system depressant and skin

irritant. Inhalation of its vapors is harmful to

the respiratory system.

8. Amyl Dimethyl PABA

A combination of PABA ester and amyl

alcohol used in sunscreens. It can cause

eczema and allergic dermatitis.

9. Barium Sulfate

A toxic and caustic chemical in many cosmetic preparations, especially hair relaxers.

10.   Behemtrimoniun Chloride

A quaternary ammonium is used as a preservative. It is a known human allergen, immune system toxin, developmental and reproductive toxin. It may cause damage to the eyes and tissue death of the mucous membranes. It is highly flammable and may be irritating to the skin.

11.   **Behemtrimonium Methosulfate**

This chemical is a human allergen and

developmental and reproductive toxin.

12.   **Benzaldehyde**

A synthetic chemical used as artificial

almond oil, and also as a preservative and

solvent. It's irritating to the eyes, skin, and

mucous membranes.

13.   **Benzalkonium Chloride**

Used as a surfactant, deodorizer, and

preservative. Health concerns include eye,

skin, and respiratory irritant. Should be

avoided, especially by individuals with asthma.

14. Benzene

This petrochemical is used as a solvent and manufacturing agent in cosmetics. It can cause depression, convulsions, coma, and death. It may be linked to leukemia. Benzene vapors can be absorbed through the skin and irritate.

15. Benzyl Alcohol

A chemical that functions as a solvent and preservative associated with allergies and organ toxicity.

16. **Boric Acid**

A Possible human endocrine (hormone)
disruptor, neurotoxin, and may be harmful
to infants.

17. **Bronopol (2-brono-2nitropopane-1,3-
Diol)**

A chemical preservative that works by
releasing formaldehyde into the product.
scores this chemical 7-9 as an overall hazard.
Other concerns include cancer and irritation
to eyes, skin, and lungs.

18. **Butylated Compounds (BHA) and (BHT)**

A chemical used as a preservative in lip, hair, makeup and other cosmetics. Health concerns include endocrine disruption, developmental and reproductive toxicity, and cancer. California's EPA Proposition 65 lists BHA as possible human carcinogen and requires warnings on products for lips.

19. **Butylene Glycol**

Functions as a humectant (attracts moisture) and fragrance for masking odors. Health concerns include irritation to eyes, skin, and lungs.

20.   Butylparaben

A member of the paraben family of preservatives.
Parabens mimic estrogen and can disrupt the
Endocrine system. Health concerns include
developmental and reproductive toxicity.

21.   Butyl Stearate

A synthetic chemical found in face creams and other
facial products. It is a possible allergen and may
cause acne.

22.   Butyrolactone

A toxic synthetic chemical used as a solvent for
Resins in cosmetics, especially nail polish.

23.   **Ceteareth (followed by any number)**

Used as a surfactant in cosmetics. Health

Concerns include enhanced skin

absorption. May contain potentially toxic

contaminants such as 1-4 dioxane.

24.   **Cetrimonium Chloride**

A quaternary ammonium compound used

as an emulsifying agent preservative and

anti-microbial. A known human allergen

and toxic to the immune system.

25.   **Cetyl Alcohol**

Considered toxic.

26. Chloroacetamide

Used as a preservative in hair, bath, and body products. This chemical is banned in France and has been found to have harmful effects on human fertility.

27. Chloroform (Methane, Trichloride)

Health concerns include endocrine disruption, cancer, organ system toxicity, and developmental and reproductive disorders. It can be irritating to skin, and lungs, and may accumulate in the body.

28.   **Coal Tar**

Used in shampoos, scalp treatments, and

Hair dyes. Coal tar is associated with

cancer of the lung, bladder, and digest

tract.

29.   **Cocamide DEA**

A human carcinogen, allergen, and

Immune system toxin.

30.   **D&C Red 30 Lake**

A synthetic dye likely sourced from

animals. Can be toxic to the human organ

system.

31. **D&C Violet 2**

A synthetic dye produced from petroleum or

coal tar. It is linked to cancer and organ

system toxicity.

32. **Dibutyl Phthalate**

Scores 10 on EWG's Database for extremely

Hazardous. Classified by the state of California

As a reproductive and developmental toxicant.

Banned in the European Union and considered an

endocrine disruptor.

33.   Diethanolamine (DEA)

Funcitons as a pH adjuster in cosmetics. Scores
10 on EWG's Database. Health hazards include
cancer, developmental, reproductive, and immune
system toxin. Other concerns include irritant to
eyes, skin, and lungs.

34.   Dimethicone/Dimeticone

Acts as a foaming agent in cosmetics and may be
the human organ system as the environment.

35.   DMDM Hydantoin

Works as a preservative in personal care products
by releasing formaldehyde. Health concerns

include cancer, irritant to eyes, skin, and lungs, and

environmental toxin.

36.   EDTA (Disodium EDTA)

Used as a chelating agent, and may be toxic to

human organ system.

37.   Ethylene Glycol

Health concerns include developmental and

reproductive toxicity. Possibly contaminated.

38.   **Ethylparaben**

Used in cosmetics as a a fragrance ingredient and

preservative. Concerns include endocrine

disruption, triggers allergies, and immune system

toxin.

39.   **Eugenol**

Used to mask odors linked to allergies, immune

system disorders, and organ system toxicity.

40.   **Ext. D&C Violet 2**

A synthetic dye produced from petroleum or

or derived from animals. Linked to allergies.

41.   FD&C Blue 1

A synthetic dye produced from petroleum or

derived from animals and linked to allergies.

42.   FD&C Green 3

A synthetic coloring ingredient possibly

derived from animals and linked to cancer.

43.   FD&C Yellow 5

A synthetic dye produced from petroleum and

toxic to organs.

44.   FD&C Yellow 6

An artificial color derived from petroleum and
toxic to organs.

45.   Fig (Ficus Carica) Extract

Functions as a skin conditioner. Health concerns
include immune system toxin and allergen.

46.   Formaldehyde

Health concerns include skin irritant that triggers
asthma, causes cancer, and pollutes the air.

47.   Fragrance/Parfum/Perfume

Defined by the FDA as a combination of chemicals

that gives each perfume or cologne (including

those used in other products) it's distinct scent.

a manufacturer has more than 3000 chemicals

available to create their proprietary or secret

formulas. These chemicals are linked to

headaches, allergies, cancer, and reproductive

disorders.

48.   Hydroquinone

A chemical used as a bleaching agent in skin

lighteners, facial moisturizers, and fade creams.

health hazards include cancer, allergen, and

immune system toxin. Toxic to the reproductive

system.

49.   **Iodopropylnyl Butylcarbanate**

Used as a preservative in cosmetics this chemical

may trigger allergies and cause contact dermatitis.

Toxic to the immune system as well as the

environment.

50.   **Imidazolidinyl Urea/Uric Acid**

A chemical that releases formaldehyde. Health

hazards include cancer, allergies, and immune

system toxin.

51.   Isobutylparaben

A member of the paraben family of preservatives.

Health concerns include estrogen mimicker, endo-

crine disruption, allergies, cancer and immune

system toxin.

52.   Isoparaffin

Derived from petroleum and toxic to human

organ system.

53.   Isopropyl Alcohol

A skin, eye and lung irritant. Vapors may cause

dizziness and/or drowsiness.

54.   Lactic Acid

Used as an exfoliant and anti-aging ingredient, and
may be derived from animals. Linked to organ
system toxicity and irritation to the eyes and skin.

55.   Lanolin

Derived from the sebaceous glands of sheep.
Toxic to the immune system, triggers allergies, and
organ system.

56.   Laureth-7

Possibly contaminated with carcinogenic 1,4
Dioxane.

57. Lead Acetate

Used in hair dyes and linked to cancer, respiratory

irritation, and reproductive toxin.

58. Methyl Methacrylate

Irritant to eyes, skin, and lungs. Toxic to the

Immune system and triggers allergies.

59. Methyparaben

A member of the paraben family of preservatives.

Parabens mimic estrogen and can act as potential

hormone disruptors. Also linked to allergies and

toxic to the immune system.

60. Mineral Oil

A liquid mixture of hydrocarbons obtained from petroleum used in baby oil, moisturizers, creams and other cosmetics. Suspected carcinogen and toxic to the immune system.

61. Monoethanolamine

Toxic to skin and respiratory tract, and may trigger allergies.

62. Nitrosamines (Diethylnitrosamines)

Linked to cancer and reproductive disorders.

63.   Nonoxynol 9,12

Possibly contaminated with ethylene oxide and

1,4-dioxane. Accumulates in wildlife.

64.   Octoxynol (9,10,11,13,40)

Irritant to eyes, skin, and lungs, and causes

hives and blistering of the skin. Contaminated

with 1,4-dioxane, ethylene oxide, and phenols.

65.   Oxybenzene

Often found in sunscreen formulations may disrupt

Normal hormone function and trigger biochemical

Or cellular changes. May cause phot allergenic

Effects and enhanced skin absorption.

66. **Padimate O**

A sunscreen agent that releases free radicals and

Causes DNA damage. An estrogen mimicker and

reproductive toxin.

67. **Para Amine Benoic Acid (PABA)**

Linked to contact dermatitis, may alter thyroid

activity, and causes cellular disorientation.

68. **Parrafin**

Derived from petroleum and linked to organ system

toxicity. Releases benzene and toluene when

heated.

69.   **PEG-100 Stearate**

Contaminated with 1,4-dioxane and ethylene

Oxide. Toxic to organs and endocrine disruptor.

70.   **Petrolatum**

A derivative of crude oil and is used in skin and

hair moisturizers and other cosmetics. Suffocates

scalp and skin, clogs pores and toxic to the human

organ system. Possibly contaminated.

71.   **Phenol**

Irritating and toxic to the respiratory system.

Toxic to the skin and kidneys.

72.   Phenoxyethanol

Widely used as a preservative in cosmetics, and is

Irritating to eyes, skin, and lungs.

73.   Placental Extract

Derived from the placenta, an organ that develops

in female mammals during pregnancy. Very likely

Derived from slaughtered animals according to

PETA. May contain waste material eliminated by

the fetus. Health concerns include infection risk,

endocrine disruption, organ system toxicity.

74.   Polyethylene Glycol (PEG7)

Strong concerns for contamination with ethylene

oxide and 1,4-dioxane, and may be toxic to organs.

75.   Polyethylene Terephthalate

Toxic to organ system, and possibly contaminated

With 1,4-dioxane. May be toxic to organs.

76.   Polysorbate 80

Possibly contaminated with 1,4-dioxane and

Ethylene glycol. Organ system toxin.

77. **Potassium Persulfate**

Triggers allergies, irritant to eyes, skin, and lungs.

Toxic to the immune system.

78. **P-phenylenediamine**

An active ingredient in hair dyes. May cause

Cancer, skin sensitivity and allergies.

79. **Potassium Hydroxide**

A caustic chemical used in hair straighteners and

relaxers. Irritant to eyes and skin, and may cause

severe burns, rashes, and hair loss. Linked to

reproductive disorders and suspected cause of

fibroid tumors.

80.   **Propyl Acetate**

Causes irritation to eyes, skin, and lungs.

81.   **Propylene Glycol**

Also known as industrial antifreeze used as a

humectant in hair and skin products as well as

Other cosmetics. Hazards include enhanced

Skin absorption, contact dermatitis, and organ

system toxicity. Irritant to eyes, skin, and lungs.

82.   **Propylparaben**

A member of the paraben family of preservatives.

Mimics estrogen, disrupts hormone system, triggers

allergies, and toxic to the immune system.

83. **Pyridine**

A toxic and flammable petrochemical formulated

Into cosmetics as a solvent. Irritating to the skin.

84. **Quaternium-15**

Linked to cancer, allergies, and immune system

toxicity. May cause developmental and

reproductive disorders, and irritating to eyes, skin,

and lungs.

85. **Resorcinol (1,3 Benzenediol, M-Hydroqinone,**
Phenylenediol)

Commonly found in hair colorants and is linked to

Cancer and immune and hormonal disorders.

86.   **Sodium Hydroxide (lye)**

The active ingredient in hair relaxers and products
That unclog your drain like Drano. It burns and
destroys organic tissue. Causes scars and deep
ulceration. Deconstructs hair and skin and is
Linked to fibroid tumors.

87.   **Sodium Laureth/Lauryl Sulfate**

Irritant to eyes, skin, and lungs, and toxic to
organs.

88.   **Sodium Metabisulfite**

Health concerns include allergies, immune system
Disorder, and eye, skin, and lung irritant.

89.   Sodium Methylparaben

Member of the paraben family of preservatives.

Mimics estrogen, hormone disruptor. Banned in the

European Union.

90.   Sodium Monoflurophosphate

Used in tooth whiteners and considered toxic to the

nervous system. Harmful if swallowed during use,

and may cause convulsions.

91.   Sulfate

A synthetic liquid made with sulfated oils used to

make synthetic soaps and detergents. Sulfates are

harmful to marine life and the environment. In

humans they cause allergic reactions, dry skin and

hair, and eye irritation.

92.   Talc

Carcinogenic and possibly contaminated with

asbestos.

93.   Teflon (PTFE)

You know it as the non-stick coating in cookware.

Part of the family of PFAS also used in makeup.

Linked to cancer and thyroid disease, especially

when used around the eyes. Avoid ingredients

with (flouro) in the name to avoid this family of

of chemicals.

94.   **Tetrasodium EDTA**

Enhances skin penetration, skin and lung irritant,

and possibly contaminated with formaldehyde.

95.   **Thimerosal**

An extremely toxic mercury-based preservative.

According to the FDA, mercury compounds are

readily absorbed through the skin and accumulate

in the body. Other concerns include cancer,

allergies, immune and reproductive system toxin.

Banned by the FDA for use in cosmetics except for

applications for the eyes.

96. Thioglycolic Acid

Used in products formulated for straightening or waving hair, and depilatory (removing hair). Possibly derived from animals and irritant to skin, eyes, and lungs. May cause skin blisters.

97. Toulene (Benzene, Toluol, Methylbenzene)

Used as a solvent in cosmetics this chemical is a potent neurotoxin. It can impair breathing, cause cancer, and irritate the eyes, skin, and lungs. Mothers exposed to vapors during pregnancy may cause damage to the fetus. Toulene is an immune system toxin and linked to blood cancer.

98.   Triclosan

Used as a preservative in personal care and home
cleaning products. Used in antibacterial soaps and
cleansers and likely contaminated with chloroform
and dioxins. An irritant to the eyes, skin, and
lungs, allergen, and disruptive to the endocrine
system. May persist and accumulate in the body.

99.   Triethanolamine

Possibly contaminated with nitrosamines and linked
To organ system toxicity.

100.   Triphenyl Phosphate

Toxic to the reproductive and immune system.

Now That You Know

"Caring for myself is not self- indulgence, it is self-preservation, and that is an act of political warfare"

–Audre Lord

This list is by no means complete of all harmful chemicals in personal care/cosmetic beauty products. This list includes the most common chemicals found in the products you use every day. It is a starting place for you to begin making healthier personal care product choices. My goal is that you know that you must take your personal-care product choices seriously because the chemicals in your cosmetics are hazardous to your health.   However, even with this new information, you may find that old habits

are hard to break. Some of the products in our

bathroom are so ubiquitous in our lives we take them

for granted. Many of which are so pervasive in the

culture we can't remember being without them.

Baby oil, for instance, is a toxic right of passage.

It's our first cosmetic, even though it is 100% mineral

oil (a derivative of petroleum). Even the fragrances

of some of these products have become a part of us

like an addiction. You can recognize the shapes and

colors of the bottles a mile away. We know exactly

where they are on the drugstore shelf, we grab the

pink and yellow bottles without thought. We slather

and rub these products on our bodies and our

children's bodies mindlessly. But I pray no more,

Pandora's box is open.

Now you know you can no longer slather, rub, and

brush these ingredients on your body unwittingly.

You have been made aware that doing so could be

exposing you and your family to hundreds of

dangerous chemicals. Many of which may cause

cancer, congenital disabilities, endocrine disruption,

neurotoxicity, and other serious health concerns.

Now you know that your headache could be the side-

effect of the celebrity-endorsed cologne you spray on

every morning. Now you know that your child's rash

that won't go away is probably due to the bubble bath

you lovingly put in their tub each night. Now you

know it's entirely possible that your seven

year old African American daughter's early

development of breast and pubic hair could be in her

hair products. Moisturizers and shampoos that

promise to give her long silky hair, may be exposing

her to chemicals with estrogenic properties that are

wreaking havoc on her hormones.

Now that you know your cosmetics may be

hazardous to your health, what are you going to do

about it? I'm sure you know that if it's going to

change it's going to be up to you and us. In the

words of the great poet June Jordan, *"We are the one's we've been waiting for."*

Here are a few suggestions that will start you on your way to a healthier cosmetic and body-care routine.

- **Read the label** and define each ingredient before choosing a cosmetic product.

- **Don't be fooled by natural claims on the front of the label.** The word natural means nothing and does not guarantee that a product is safe.

- **Look for plant-based products.** The USDA Organic label or "Made with Organic Ingredients" indicate products mostly made of plants.

- **Take a good hard and honest look** at what's in your bathroom and makeup bag and determine if and how much you are exposing you and your family to harmful chemicals.

- **As soon as possible eliminate and replace** the most toxic products

- **Less is safer.** Throw out expired and old products.

- **Decreasing the number of products** in your routine decreases harmful exposure. Think about it, do you need bar soap and shower gel or body lotion and hand lotion? Do your research and opt for the cleanest least complicated solution to your needs.

- **Visit your local natural product or health food stores** to familiarize yourself with safer alternatives.

The buyers work hard to stock their shelves with clean and healthy products. Talk to staff members. The staff in natural product stores are very committed to natural and healthy lifestyles and are very eager to share their knowledge. However, take nothing for granted and read and verify the ingredients of any product recommendations, no matter where you buy it.

- **Consider making your own products**. There are numerous books and internet pages filled with natural product recipes that use simple kitchen ingredients.

- **Seek out hand made products on the internet.** There are plenty of healthy choices.

- **Commit to a healthy lifestyle.** Begin the journey, seek, and you will find the answers. Research and learn as much as you can.

- **Demand clean, healthy products.** Black women spend more money on hair and personal care products than any other demographic to the tune of $7Billion a year. You better believe big and small corporations will sell you down the river for a profit and could care less if they are exposing you to toxic chemicals. They are not going to change unless you short their money. Collectively we have the power to make this change.

- **Use every resource available.**

- **Greensistah.com** is a website dedicated to providing awareness, coaching and empowerment to help you transform your lifestyle to one that is healing to your mind, body, and spirit.

- **Detox Me is an app created by Silent Spring Institute.** Available on your smartphone, it walks you through simple, researched-based tips to reduce exposure to toxic chemicals where you live, work, and play.

- **Healthy living is an app created by The Environmental Working Group (EWG),** where there are ratings for more than 120,000 personal care and food products. You can scan the item, check its hazard score, and make a healthier educated choice.

Take Inventory

- How many of the "Nasty 100" are you exposing yourself to?

- How many products do you use daily?

- How many times a day do you use them?

- Are you experiencing any of the harmful effect of the chemicals you are exposed to?

- How many fragrances are you and your family exposed to daily?

Become a Cosmetic Label Snob!

Demand and purchase only the best products available, and snub anything less. Your health and health of the Next seven generations depend on how committed you become to eliminating toxic ingredients from your personal care routine. Its going to be totally up to you. There is no government agency regulating what goes into your cosmetics and the manufacturers are going to keep doing what makes them huge profits at the expense of your health.

Glossary of Terms

Allergen

A substance capable of triggering a response that starts in the immune system and results in an allergic reaction.

Anti-aging

A product or technique designed to prevent the appearance of getting older.

Carcinogenic

Having the potential to cause cancer.

Caustic chemical

Describes a chemical that is able to burn living tissue or other substances.

Contact dermatitis

A red, itchy rash caused by direct contact with a substance or an allergic reaction to it.

Contamination

Being made impure by pollution or poisoning.

Cosmetic

A product applied to the hair, skin, or nails to improve one's appearance.

Depilatory

Used to remove unwanted hair

Endocrine disruption

Chemicals that can interfere with endocrine (or hormonal) systems at certain doses. These disruptions

can cause cancerous tumors, birth defects, and other
developmental disorders.

Endocrine system

A network of glands in your body that make the hormones
and help the cells communicate with each other.

Enhanced skin absorption

A route where substance can enter the body and blood
stream through the skin.

Environmental Working Group (EWG)

A non-profit that empowers people to live healthier lives
in a healthier environment. EWG's database rates more
than 70,000 personal care ingredients and products for
safety.

Estrogen

A group of steroid hormones which promote the development and maintenance of female characteristics of the body.

Estrogen mimickers

A substance that imitates estrogen

Exfoliate

The process of removing dead skin cells from the surface of the skin using a chemical, granular substance, or exfoliation tool.

FDA

An abbreviation for the Food & Drug Administration. The FDA is responsible for protecting the public health by ensuring the safety, efficacy, and security of human and veterinary drugs, biological products, and medical

devices; and by ensuring the safety of our nation's food

supply, cosmetics, and products that emit radiation.

Free Radicals

Unpaired electrons due to the oxidative stress that

Occurs when oxygen molecules split into single atoms.

Hormones

A regulatory substance produced in an organism and

transported in fluid such as blood to stimulate specific

cells or tissues into action.

Humectant

A moisturizing agent found in lotions, shampoos, creams,

and other beauty and cosmetic products for hair and skin

to retain moisture.

Immune System

The body's defense against infection, attacks germs, and

Helps keep us healthy.

Natural

Existing in or caused by nature. Not caused or made by

humankind.

Neurotoxin

Toxins that are destructive to nerve tissue

Nitrosamines

Toxic compounds

PETA

People for the ethical treatment of animals, is the largest

animal rights organization in the world.

Petrochemical

Chemical substances derived as the result of refining petroleum.

Photo sensitivity

An immune system reaction that is triggered by sunlight.

Placenta

An organ that develops in the uterus during pregnancy.

Plasticizers

Additives that increase the plasticity or decrease the viscosity of a material or substance.

Preservative

In cosmetics, a substance used to protect the products against decay, discoloration, or spoilage.

Reproductive/developmental system

The system of organs and parts which function in reproduction consisting in the male especially of the testes, penis, seminal vesicles, prostate and urethra. In the female it includes the ovaries, fallopian tubes, uterus, vagina, and vulva.

Sebaceous Glands

A small gland in the skin which secretes a lubricating oily matter (sebum) into the hair follicles to lubricate the hair and the skin.

Silent Spring Institute

The leading scientific research organization dedicated to uncovering the links between chemicals in our everyday environment and women's health, with a focus on breast cancer prevention.

Solvent

A chemical that dissolves other substances.

Surfactant

Surfactants are compounds that lower the surface tension between two liquids, between a gas and a liquid, or between a liquid and a solid. Surfactants may act as detergents, wetting agents, emulsifiers, foaming agents, and dispersants.

Toxin

A poisonous substance produced within living cells or Organisms.

Resources

Websites:

Greensistah.com

Ewg.org

cosmeticsdatabase.com

safecosmetics.org

nottoopretty.org

Leapingbunny.org

womensvoics.org

silentspringinstitute.org

Books

There's Lead in Your Lipstick, Gillian Deacon, Penguin Books, 2010.

Ecoholic, Adria Vasil, Random House Canada, 2007.

No More Dirty Looks: The Truth About Your Beauty Products and the Ultimate Guide to Safe and Clean Cosmetics, Siobhan O'Connor & Alexandra Spunt, Perseus Books, 2010.

Toxic Beauty: How Cosmetics and Personal Care Products Endanger Your Health. And What You Can Do About It, Samuel S. Epstein & Randall Fitzgerald, Ben Bella Books, 2009.

Not Just A Pretty Face, Stacey Malkan, New Society Publishers, 2007.

Drop-dead Gorgeous, Kim Erikson, Contemporary

Books, 2002.

Home Safe Home, Debra Lynn Dadd, Tarcher Inc, 2005.

*Better Basics for the Home: Simple Solutions for Less

Toxic Living*, Annie Berthold Bond, Three Rivers Press,

1999.

Videos

The Story of Cosmetics, Annie Leonard

available on youtube

Stink the Movie, A Documentary by John Whelan;

stinkmovie.com

Notes

About the Author

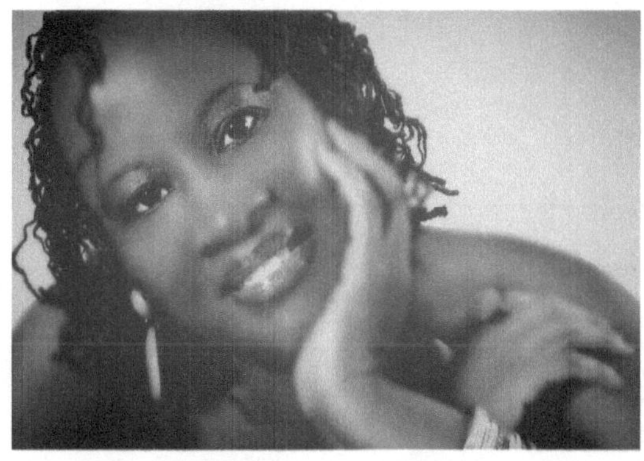

Willette Monk

Graduate of Christopher Newport University

Founder of the GreenSistah™Project

Certified Green/Sustainable Lifestyle Coach

Licensed Esthetician Hair loss Consultant

Master Cosmetic Formulator

Contact Willette at: greensistah@greensistah.com